Mediterr
Recipe Co

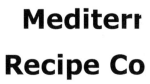

CW00448618

Quick and Easy Recipes

To Weight Loss

Ben Cooper

© Copyright 2020 - All rights reserved.

The content contained within this book may not be reproduced, duplicated or transmitted without direct written permission from the author or the publisher.

Under no circumstances will any blame or legal responsibility be held against the publisher, or author, for any damages, reparation, or monetary loss due to the information contained within this book. Either directly or indirectly.

Legal Notice:

This book is copyright protected. This book is only for personal use. You cannot amend, distribute, sell, use, quote or paraphrase any part, or the content within this book, without the consent of the author or publisher.

Disclaimer Notice:

Please note the information contained within this document is for educational and entertainment purposes only. All effort has been executed to present accurate, up to date, and reliable, complete information. No warranties of any kind are declared or implied. Readers acknowledge that the author is not engaging in the rendering of legal, financial, medical or professional advice. The content within this book has been derived from various sources. Please consult a licensed professional before attempting any techniques outlined in this book.

By reading this document, the reader agrees that under no circumstances is the author responsible for any losses, direct or indirect, which are incurred as a result of the use of information contained within this document, including, but not limited to, — errors, omissions, or inaccuracies.

Table of Contents

Hummus with Ground Lamb

Preparation Time: 10 minutes
Cooking Time: 15 minute
Servings: 8

Ingredients:

10 oz. hummus
12 oz. lamb meat, ground
½ cup pomegranate seeds
¼ cup parsley, chopped
1 tbsp. olive oil
Pita chips for serving

Directions:

1.Heat a pan with the oil over medium-high heat, add the meat, and brown for 15 minutes stirring often.

2.Spread the hummus on a platter, spread the ground lamb all over, and spread the pomegranate seeds and the parsley and serve with pita chips.

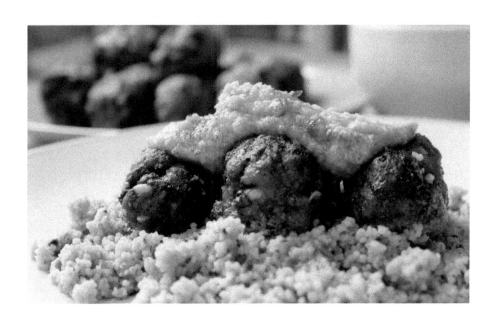

Wrapped Plums Preparation

Preparation Time: 5 minutes
Cooking Time: 0 minutes
Servings: 8

Ingredients:

2 oz. prosciutto, cut into 16 pieces
4 plums, quartered
1 tbsp. chives, chopped
A pinch of red pepper flakes, crushed

Directions:

1.Wrap each plum quarter in a prosciutto slice, arrange them all on a platter, sprinkle the chives and pepper flakes all over and serve.

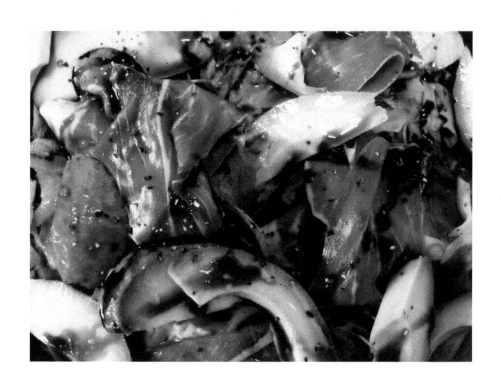

Cucumber Sandwich Bites

Preparation Time: 5 minutes
Cooking Time: 0 minutes
Servings: 12

Ingredients:

1 cucumber, sliced
8 slices whole wheat bread
2 tbsp. cream cheese, soft
1 tbsp. chives, chopped
¼ cup avocado, peeled, pitted and mashed
1 tsp. mustard
Salt and black pepper to the taste

Directions:

1.Spread the mashed avocado on each bread slice, also spread the rest of the ingredients except the cucumber slices.

2.Divide the cucumber slices on the bread slices, cut each slice in thirds, arrange on a platter and serve as an appetizer.

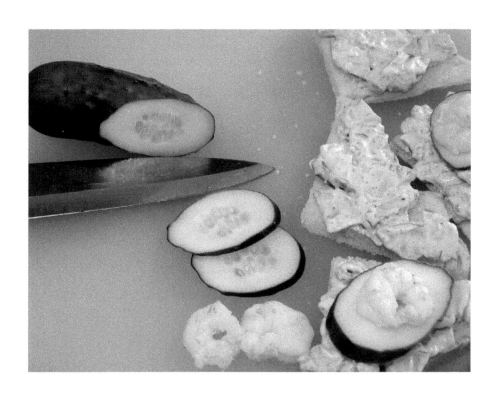

Cucumber Rolls

Preparation Time: 5 minutes
Cooking Time: 0 minutes
Servings: 6

Ingredients:

1 big cucumber, sliced lengthwise
1 tbsp. parsley, chopped
8 oz. canned tuna, drained and mashed
Salt and black pepper to the taste
1 tsp. lime juice

Directions:

1.Arrange cucumber slices on a working surface, divide the rest of the ingredients, and roll.

2.Arrange all the rolls on a platter and serve as an appetizer.

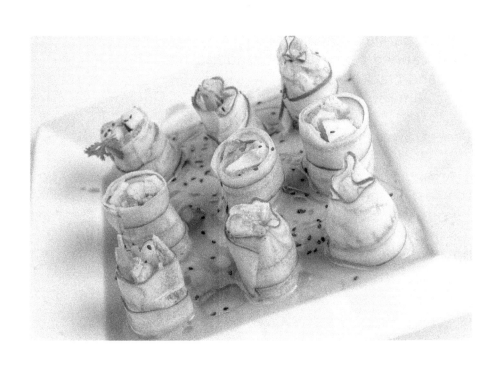

Olives and Cheese Stuffed Tomatoes

Preparation Time: 10 minutes
Cooking Time: 0 minutes
Servings: 24

Ingredients:

24 cherry tomatoes, top cut off and insides scooped out
2 tbsp. olive oil
¼ tsp. red pepper flakes
½ cup feta cheese, crumbled
2 tbsp. black olive paste
¼ cup mint, torn

Directions:

1.In a bowl, mix the olives paste with the rest of the ingredients except the cherry tomatoes and whisk. Stuff the cherry tomatoes with this mix, arrange them all on a platter and serve as an appetizer.

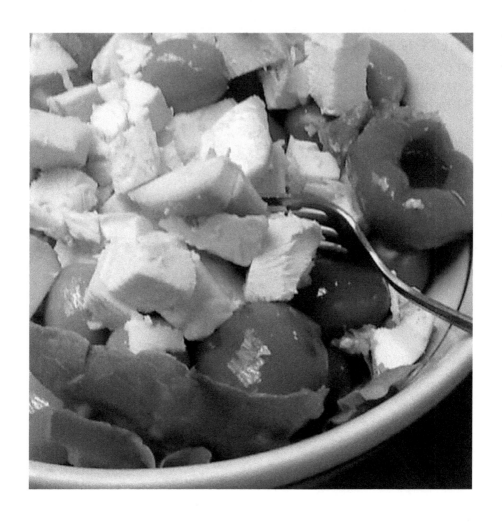

Tomato Salsa

Preparation Time: 5 minutes
Cooking Time: 0 minutes
Servings: 6

Ingredients:

1 garlic clove, minced
4 tbsp. olive oil
5 tomatoes, cubed
1 tbsp. balsamic vinegar
¼ cup basil, chopped
1 tbsp. parsley, chopped
1 tbsp. chives, chopped
Salt and black pepper to the taste
Pita chips for serving

Directions:

1.In a bowl, mix the tomatoes with the garlic and the rest of the ingredients except the pita chips, stir, divide into small cups and serve with the pita chips on the side.

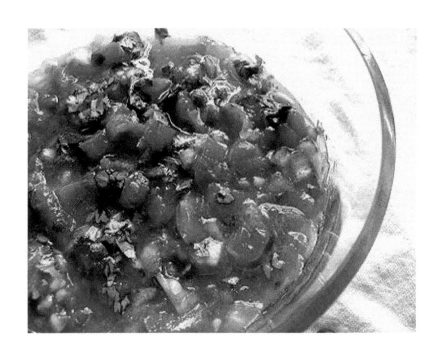

Chili Mango and Watermelon Salsa

Preparation Time: 5 minutes
Cooking Time: 0 minutes
Servings: 12

Ingredients:

1 red tomato, chopped
Salt and black pepper to the taste
1 cup watermelon, seedless, peeled and cubed
1 red onion, chopped
2 mangos, peeled and chopped
2 chili peppers, chopped
¼ cup cilantro, chopped
3 tbsp. lime juice
Pita chips for serving

Directions:

1.In a bowl, mix the tomato with the watermelon, the onion and the rest of the ingredients except the pita chips and toss well.

2.Divide the mix into small cups and serve with pita chips on the side.

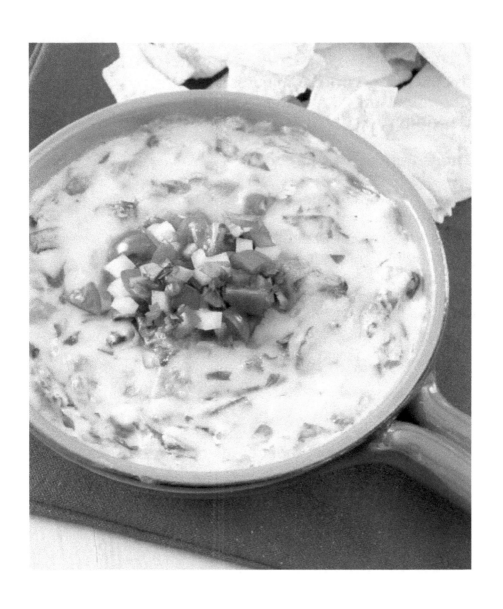

Creamy Spinach and Shallots Dip

Preparation Time: 10 minutes
Cooking Time: 0 minutes
Servings: 4

Ingredients:

1 lb. spinach, roughly chopped
2 shallots, chopped
2 tbsp. mint, chopped
¾ cup cream cheese, soft
Salt and black pepper to the taste

Directions:

1.In a blender, combine the spinach with the shallots and the rest of the ingredients, and pulse well.

2. Divide into small bowls and serve as a party dip.

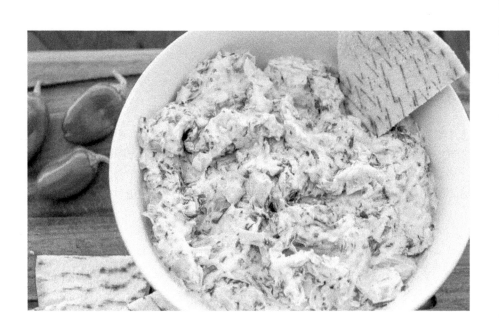

Feta Artichoke

Preparation Time: 10 minutes

Cooking Time: 30 minutes

Servings: 8

Ingredients:

8 oz. artichoke hearts, drained and quartered
¾ cup basil, chopped
¾ cup green olives, pitted and chopped
1 cup parmesan cheese, grated
5 oz. feta cheese, crumbled

Directions:

1.In your food processor, mix the artichokes with the basil and the rest of the ingredients, pulse well, and transfer to a baking dish.

2.Introduce in the oven, bake at 375° F for 30 minutes and serve as a party dip.

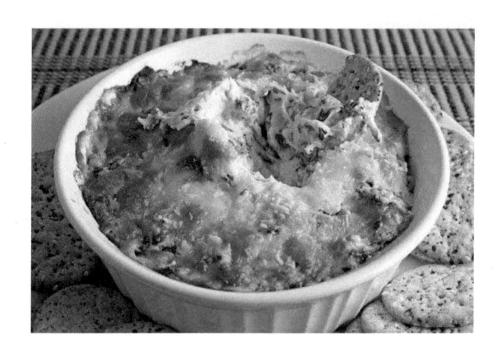

Chickpeas and Beets Mix

Preparation Time: 10 minutes
Cooking Time: 25 minutes
Servings: 4

Ingredients:

3 tablespoons capers, drained and chopped Juice of 1 lemon
Zest of 1 lemon, grated
1 red onion, chopped
3 tablespoons olive oil
14 ounces canned chickpeas, drained 8 ounces beets, peeled and cubed
1 tablespoon parsley, chopped
Salt and pepper to the taste

Directions:

1.Heat a pan with the oil over medium heat, add the onion, lemon zest, lemon juice and the capers and sauté for 5 minutes.

2.Add the rest of the ingredients, stir and cook over medium-low heat for 20 minutes more.

3.Divide the mix between plates and serve as a side dish.

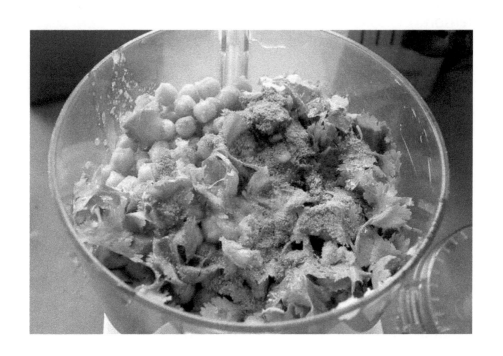

Creamy Sweet Potatoes Mix

Preparation Time: 10 minutes
Cooking Time: 1 hour
Servings: 4

Ingredients:

4 tablespoons olive oil
1 garlic clove, minced
4 medium sweet potatoes, pricked with a fork
1 red onion, sliced
3 ounces baby spinach
Zest and juice of 1 lemon
A small bunch dill, chopped
1 and ½ tablespoons Greek yogurt
2 tablespoons tahini paste
Salt and black pepper to the taste

Directions:

1.Put the potatoes on a baking sheet lined with parchment paper, introduce in the oven at 350 degrees F and cook them for 1 hour.

2.Peel the potatoes, cut them into wedges and put them in a bowl.

3.Add the garlic, the oil and the rest of the ingredients, toss, divide the mix between plates and serve.

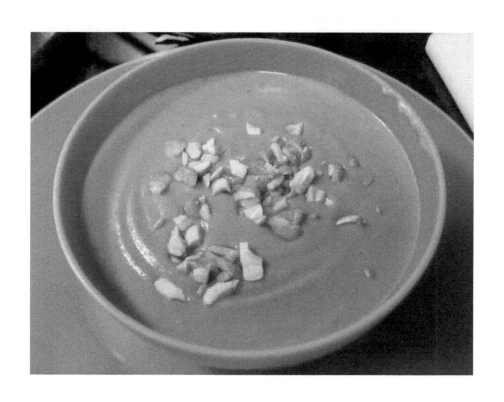

Cabbage and Mushrooms Mix

Preparation Time: 10 minutes
Cooking Time: 15 minutes
Servings: 2

Ingredients:

1 yellow onion, sliced
2 tablespoons olive oil
1 tablespoon balsamic vinegar
½ pound white mushrooms, sliced
1 green cabbage head, shredded
4 spring onions, chopped
Salt and black pepper to the taste

Directions:

1.Heat a pan with the oil over medium heat, add the yellow onion and the spring onions and cook for 5 minutes.

2.Add the rest of the ingredients, cook everything for 10 minutes, divide between plates and serve.

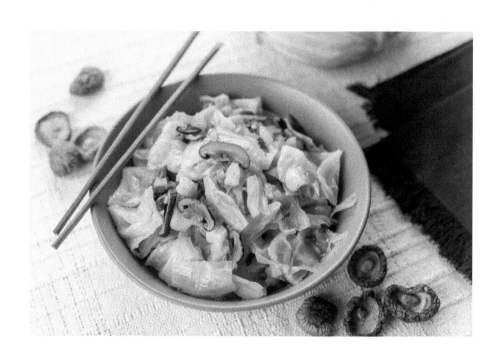

Lemon Mushroom Rice

Preparation Time: 10 minutes
Cooking Time: 30 minutes
Servings: 4

Ingredients:

2 cups chicken stock
1 yellow onion, chopped
½ pound white mushrooms, sliced
2 garlic cloves, minced
8 ounces wild rice
Juice and zest of 1 lemon
1 tablespoon chives, chopped
6 tablespoons goat cheese, crumbled
Salt and black pepper to the taste

Directions:

1.Heat a pot with the stock over medium heat, add the rice, onion and the rest of the ingredients except the chives and the cheese, bring to a simmer and cook for 25 minutes.

2.Add the remaining ingredients, cook everything for 5 minutes, divide between plates and serve as a side dish.

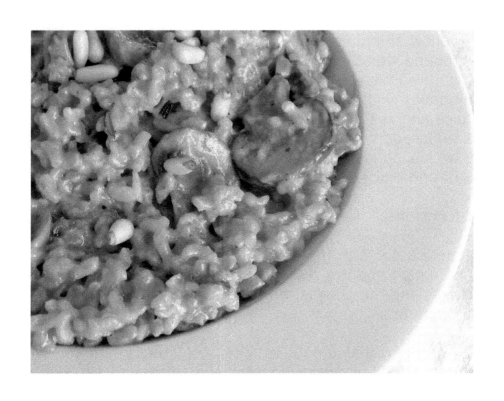

Paprika and Chives Potatoes

Preparation Time: 10 minutes
Cooking Time: 1 hour and 8 minutes
Servings: 4

Ingredients:

4 potatoes, scrubbed and pricked with a fork
1 tablespoon olive oil
1 celery stalk, chopped 2 tomatoes, chopped
1 teaspoon sweet paprika
Salt and black pepper to the taste
2 tablespoons chives, chopped

Directions:

1.Arrange the potatoes on a baking sheet lined with parchment paper, introduce in the oven and bake at 350 degrees F for 1 hour.

2.Cool the potatoes down, peel and cut them into larger cubes.

3.Heat a pan with the oil over medium heat, add the celery and the tomatoes and sauté for 2 minutes.

4.Add the potatoes and the rest of the ingredients, toss, cook everything for 6 minutes, divide the mix between plates and serve as a side dish.

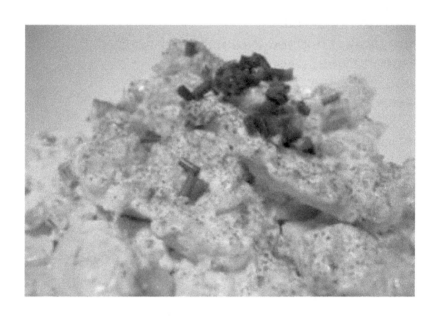

Bulgur, Kale and Cheese Mix

Preparation Time: 10 minutes
Cooking Time: 10 minutes
Servings: 6

Ingredients:

4 ounces bulgur
4 ounces kale, chopped
1 tablespoon mint, chopped
3 spring onions, chopped
1 cucumber, chopped
A pinch of allspice, ground
2 tablespoons olive oil
Zest and juice of ½ lemon
4 ounces feta cheese, crumbled

Directions:

1.Put bulgur in a bowl, cover with hot water, aside for 10 minutes and fluff with a fork.

2.Heat a pan with the oil over medium heat, add the onions and the allspice and cook for 3 minutes.

3.Add the bulgur and the rest of the ingredients, cook everything for 5-6 minutes more, divide between plates and serve.

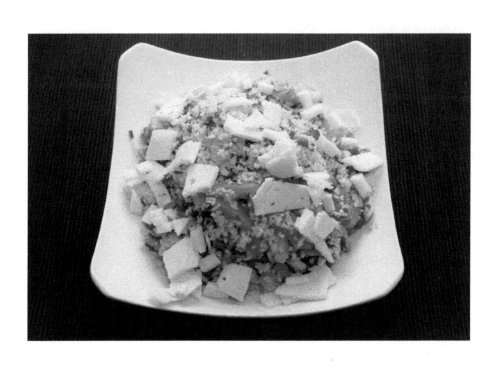

Spicy Green Beans Mix

Preparation Time: 5 minutes
Cooking Time: 15 minutes
Servings: 4

Ingredients:

4 teaspoons olive oil
1 garlic clove, minced
½ teaspoon hot paprika
¾ cup veggie stock
1 yellow onion, sliced
1 pound green beans, trimmed and halved
½ cup goat cheese, shredded
2 teaspoon balsamic vinegar

Directions:

1.Heat a pan with the oil over medium heat, add the garlic, stir and cook for 1 minute.

2.Add the green beans and the rest of the ingredients, toss, cook everything for 15 minutes more, divide between plates and serve as a side dish.

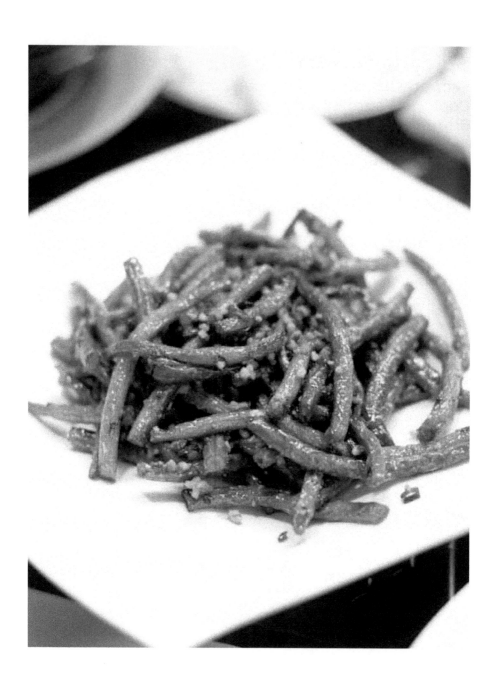

Beans and Rice

Preparation Time: 10 minutes
Cooking Time: 55 minutes
Servings: 6

Ingredients:

1 tablespoon olive oil
1 yellow onion, chopped
2 celery stalks, chopped
2 garlic cloves, minced
2 cups brown rice
1 and ½ cup canned black beans, rinsed and drained
4 cups water
Salt and black pepper to the taste

Directions:

1.Heat a pan with the oil over medium heat, add the celery, garlic and the onion, stir and cook for 10 minutes.

2.Add the rest of the ingredients, stir, bring to a simmer and cook over medium heat for 45 minutes.

3.Divide between plates and serve.

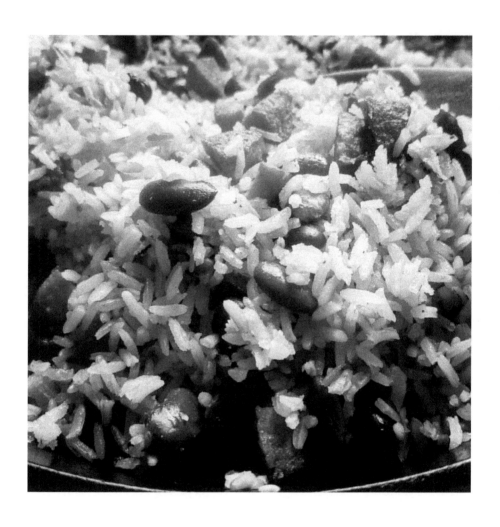

Tomato and Millet Mix

Preparation Time: 10 minutes
Cooking Time: 20 minutes
Servings: 6

Ingredients:

3 tablespoons olive oil
1 cup millet
2 spring onions, chopped
2 tomatoes, chopped
½ cup cilantro, chopped
1 teaspoon chili paste
6 cups cold water
½ cup lemon juice
Salt and black pepper to the taste

Directions:

1.Heat a pan with the oil over medium heat, add the millet, stir and cook for 4 minutes.

2.Add the water, salt and pepper, stir, and bring a simmer over medium heat cook for 15 minutes.

3.Add the rest of the ingredients, toss, divide the mix between plates and serve as a side dish.

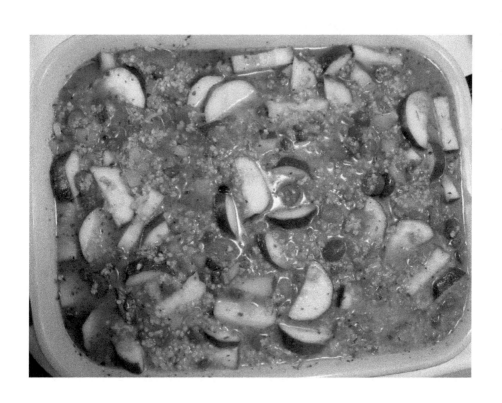

Quinoa and Greens Salad

Preparation Time: 10 minutes
Cooking Time: 0 minutes
Servings: 4

Ingredients:

1 cup quinoa, cooked
1 medium bunch collard greens, chopped
4 tablespoons walnuts, chopped
2 tablespoons balsamic vinegar
4 tablespoons tahini paste
4 tablespoons cold water
A pinch of salt and black pepper
1 tablespoon olive oil

Directions:

1.In a bowl, mix the tahini with the water and vinegar and whisk.

2.In a bowl, mix the quinoa with the rest of the ingredients and the tahini dressing, toss, divide the mix between plates and serve as a side dish.

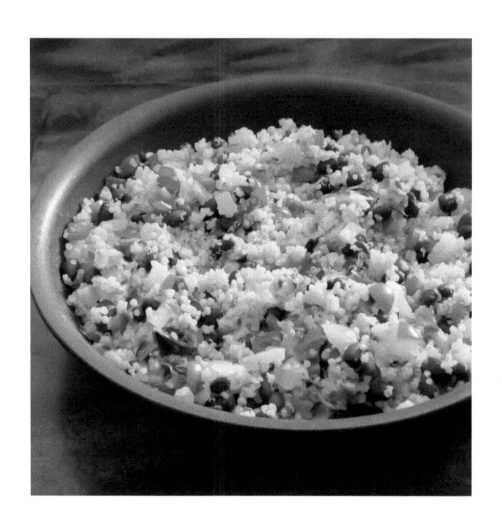

Veggies and Avocado Dressing
Preparation Time: 10 minutes
Cooking Time: 0 minutes
Servings: 4

Ingredients:

3 tablespoons pepitas, roasted
3 cups water
2 tablespoons cilantro, chopped
4 tablespoons parsley, chopped
1 and ½ cups corn
1 cup radish, sliced
2 avocados, peeled, pitted and chopped
2 mangos, peeled and chopped
3 tablespoons olive oil
4 tablespoons Greek yogurt
1 teaspoons balsamic vinegar
2 tablespoons lime juice
Salt and black pepper to the taste

Directions:

1.In your blender, mix the olive oil with avocados, salt, pepper, lime juice, the yogurt and the vinegar and pulse.

2.In a bowl, mix the pepitas with the cilantro, parsley and the rest of the ingredients, and toss.

3.Add the avocado dressing, toss, divide the mix between plates and serve as a side dish.

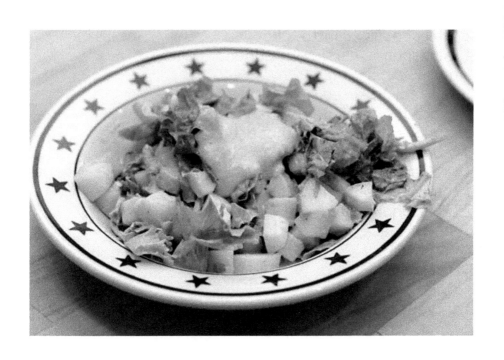

Guacamole

Preparation Time: 10 minutes
Cooking Time: 0 minutes
Servings: 4

Ingredients:

3 avocados - peeled, seeded and mashed
1 lime, juiced
1 teaspoon salt
1/2 cup diced onion
3 tablespoons chopped fresh coriander
2 Roma tomatoes, diced
1 teaspoon chopped garlic
1 pinch of ground cayenne pepper (optional)

Directions:

1.Puree avocados, lime juice, and salt in a medium bowl.

2.Stir in the onion, coriander, tomatoes, and garlic. Stir in the cayenne pepper.

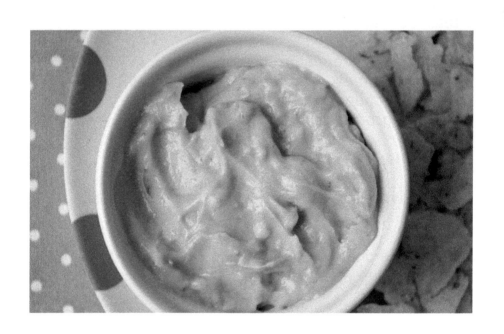

Sugar-coated Pecans

Preparation Time: 15 minutes
Cooking Time: 1 hour
Servings: 12

Ingredients:

1 egg white
1 tablespoon water
1 pound pecan halves
1 cup white sugar
3/4 teaspoon salt
1/2 teaspoon ground cinnamon

Directions:

1.Preheat the oven to 120 ° C (250 ° F). Grease a baking tray.

2.In a bowl, whisk the egg whites and water until frothy. Combine the sugar, salt, and cinnamon in another bowl.

3.Add the pecans to the egg whites and stir to cover the nuts.

4.Remove the nuts and mix them with the sugar until well covered. Spread the nuts on the prepared baking sheet.

5.Bake for 1 hour at 250 ° F (120 ° C). Stir every 15 minutes.

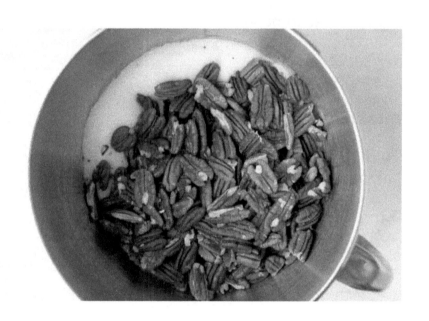

Southwestern Egg Rolls
Preparation Time: 20 minutes
Cooking Time: 20 minutes
Servings: 5

Ingredients:

2 tablespoons vegetable oil
1/2 chicken fillet, skinless
2 tablespoons chopped green onion
2 tablespoons chopped red pepper
1/3 cup frozen corn kernels
1/4 cup black beans, rinsed and drained
2 tablespoons chopped frozen spinach, thawed and drained
2 tablespoons diced jalapeño peppers
1/2 tablespoon chopped fresh parsley
1/2 c. ground cumin
1/2 teaspoon chili powder
1/3 teaspoon salt
1 pinch of ground cayenne pepper
3/4 cup of grated Monterey Jack cheese
5 flour tortillas (6 inches)
1 liter of oil for frying

Directions:

1.Rub 1 tablespoon of vegetable oil on the chicken fillet.

2.Cook the chicken in a medium-sized saucepan over medium heat for about 5 minutes per side until the meat is no longer pink and the juice is clear.

3.Remove from heat and set aside.

4.Heat 1 tablespoon of remaining vegetable oil in a medium-sized saucepan over medium heat. Stir in the green onion and red pepper. Boil and stir for 5 minutes, until soft.

5.Cut the diced chicken and mix in the pan with the onion and red pepper. Mix corn, black beans, spinach, jalapeño pepper, parsley, cumin, chili powder, salt, and cayenne pepper.

6.Boil and stir for 5 minutes, until everything is well mixed and soft. Remove from heat and stir in Monterey Jack cheese until it melts.

7..Wrap the tortillas with a clean, slightly damp cloth — microwave at maximum power, about 1 minute, or until it is hot and malleable.

8..Pour equal amounts of the mixture into each tortilla.

9..Fold the ends of the tortillas and wrap the mixture well. Safe with toothpicks. Arrange in a medium-sized dish, cover with plastic, and place in the freezer. Freeze for at least 4 hours.

10.Heat the oil in a deep frying pan to 190° C for frying. Bake frozen stuffed tortillas for 10 minutes or until golden brown. Drain on paper towels before serving.

Annie's Salsa Chips with Fruit & Cinnamon

Preparation Time: 15 minutes
Cooking Time: 15 minutes
Servings: 10

Ingredients:

2 Golden Delicious apples - peeled, seeded and diced
8 grams of raspberry
2 kiwis, peeled and diced
1 pound of strawberries
2 tablespoons of white sugar
1 tablespoon of brown sugar
3 tablespoons canned fruit Flour cooking aerosol
Flour tortillas
2 tablespoons cinnamon sugar

Directions:

1.Combine kiwi, Golden Delicious apples, raspberries, strawberries, white sugar, brown sugar, and canned fruit in a large bowl. Cover and put in the fridge for at least 15 minutes.

2.Preheat the oven to 175 ° C (350 ° F).
Cover one side of each flour tortilla with a cooking spray.

3.Cut into segments and place them in one layer on a large baking sheet. Sprinkle the quarters with the desired amount of cinnamon sugar. Spray again with cooking spray.

4.Bake in the preheated oven for 8 to 10 minutes.
Repeat this with the other tortilla quarters.

5.Cool for approximately 15 minutes. Serve with a
mixture of
fresh fruit.

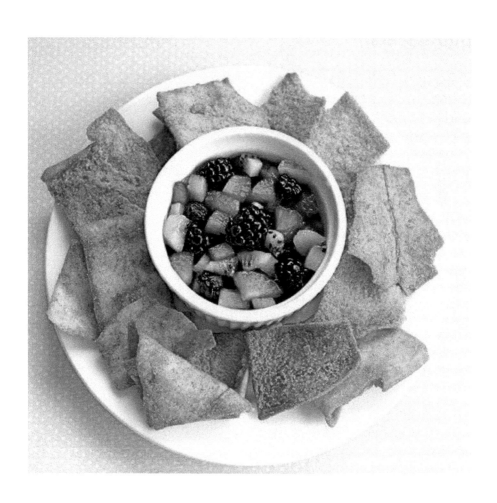

Boneless Buffalo Wings

Preparation Time: 10 minutes
Cooking Time: 15 minutes
Servings: 3

Ingredients:

Frying oil
1 cup unbleached flour
2 teaspoons of salt
1/2 teaspoon ground black pepper
1/2 teaspoon cayenne pepper
1/4 teaspoon garlic powder
1/2 teaspoon bell pepper
1 egg
1 cup of milk
3 boneless chicken fillets, skinless, cut into 1/2 inch strips
1/4 cup hot pepper sauce
1 tablespoon butter

Directions:

1.Heat the oil in a frying pan or large saucepan.

2.Mix the flour, salt, black pepper, cayenne pepper, garlic powder, and bell pepper in a large bowl. Beat the egg and milk in a small bowl.

3Dip each piece of chicken in the egg mixture and then roll it into the flour mixture.

4.Repeat the process so that each piece of chicken is doubled. Cool the breaded chicken for 20 minutes.

5.Fry chicken in hot oil, in batches. Cook until the outside is well browned and the juice is clear, 5 to 6 minutes per batch.

6.Mix the hot sauce and butter in a small bowl. Heat the sauce in the microwave on high to melt, 20 to 30 seconds. Pour the sauce over the cooked chicken; mix well.

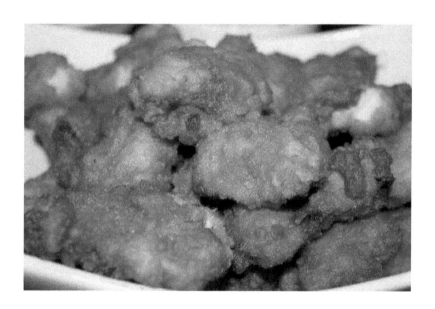

Jalapeño Popper Spread

Preparation Time: 10 minutes
Cooking Time: 3 minutes
Servings: 32

Ingredients:

2 packets of cream cheese, softened
1 cup mayonnaise
1 (4-gram) can chopped green peppers, drained
2 grams diced jalapeño peppers, canned, drained
1 cup grated Parmesan cheese

Directions:

1.In a large bowl, mix cream cheese and mayonnaise until smooth. Stir the bell peppers and jalapeño peppers.

2.Pour the mixture into a microwave oven and sprinkle with Parmesan cheese. Microwave on maximum power, about 3 minutes.

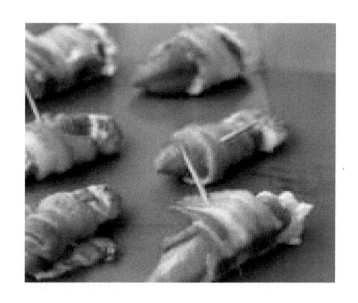

Brown Sugar Smokies

Preparation Time: 10 minutes
Cooking Time: 10 minutes
Servings: 12

Ingredients:

1 pound bacon
1 (16 ounces) package little smoky sausages
1 cup brown sugar, or to taste

Directions:

1.Preheat the oven to 175 ° C (350 ° F).

2.Cut the bacon in three and wrap each strip around a little sausage.

3.Place sausages wrapped on wooden skewers, several to one place the kebabs on a baking sheet and sprinkle generously with brown sugar.

4.Bake until the bacon is crispy, and the brown sugar has melted.

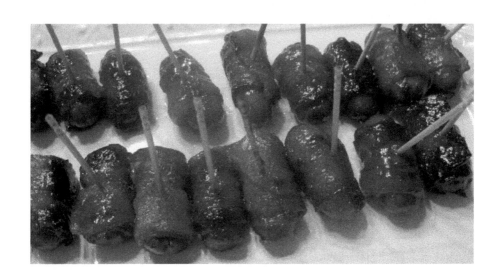

Pita Chips

Preparation Time: 10 minutes
Cooking Time: 8 minutes
Servings: 24

Ingredients:

12 slices of pita bread
1/2 cup of olive oil
1/2 teaspoon ground black pepper
1 teaspoon garlic salt
1/2 teaspoon dried basil
1 teaspoon dried chervil

Directions:

1.Preheat the oven to 200 degrees C (400 degrees F).

2.Cut each pita bread into 8 triangles. Place the triangles on the baking sheet.

3.Combine oil, pepper, salt, basil, and chervil in a small bowl. Brush each triangle with the oil mixture.

4.Bake in the preheated oven for about 7 minutes or until light brown and crispy.

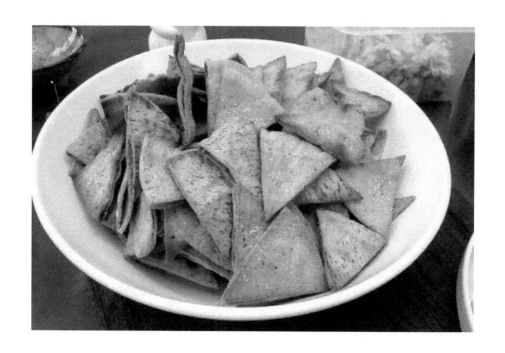

Hot Spinach, Artichoke & Chili Dip

Preparation Time: 10 minutes
Cooking Time: 30 minutes
Servings: 10

Ingredients:

2 (8 oz.) packages of cream cheese, softened
1/2 cup of mayonnaise
1 can (4.5 oz.) chopped green pepper, drained
1 cup of freshly grated Parmesan cheese
1 jar (12 oz.) marinated artichoke hearts, drained and chopped
1/4 cup canned chopped jalapeño peppers, drained
1 can of chopped spinach frozen, thawed and drained

Directions:

1.Preheat the oven to 175 ° C (350 ° F).

2.Mix the cream cheese and mayonnaise in a bowl. Stir the green peppers, parmesan cheese, artichokes, peppers, and spinach.

3.Pour the mixture into a baking dish.

4.Bake in the preheated oven until light brown, about 30 minutes.

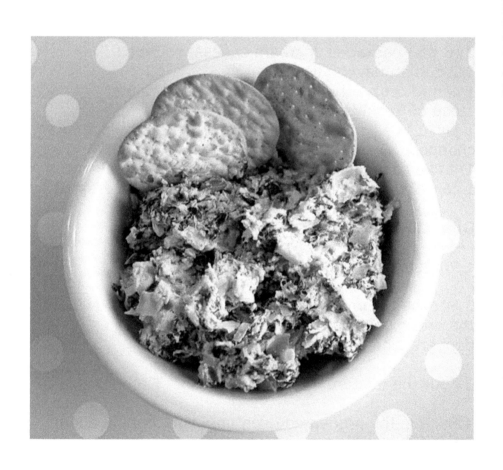

Fruit Dip
Preparation Time: 5 minutes
Cooking Time: 0 minutes
Servings: 12

Ingredients:

1 (8-oz.) package cream cheese, softened
1 (7-oz.) jar marshmallow crème

Directions:

1.Use an electric mixer to combine the cream cheese and marshmallow Beat until everything is well mixed.

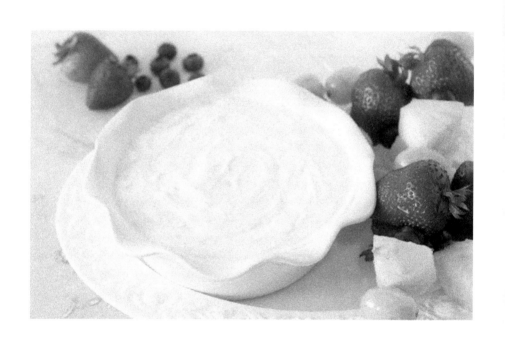

Banana & Tortilla Snacks

Preparation Time: 5 minutes
Cooking Time: 0 minutes
Servings: 1

Ingredients:

1 flour tortilla (6 inches)
2 tablespoons peanut butter
1 tablespoon honey
1 banana
2 tablespoons raisins

Directions:

1.Lay the tortilla flat. Spread peanut butter and honey on the tortilla.

2.Place the banana in the middle and sprinkle the raisins.

3.Wrap and serve.

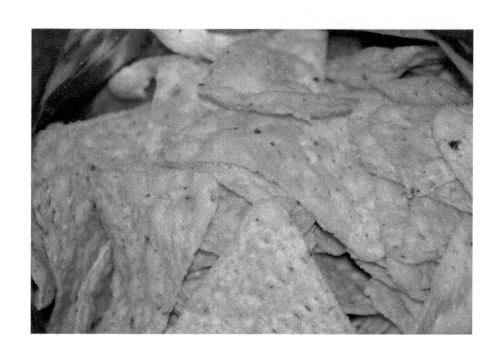

Wonton Snacks

Preparation Time: 20 minutes
Cooking Time: 12 minutes
Servings: 48

Ingredients:

2 pounds of ground pork
2 stalks of celery
2 carrots
2 cloves of garlic
1 small onion
1 (8-gram) can water chestnuts
1/2 cup of Thai peanut sauce prepared
1 package (14-oz.) wonton wraps

Directions:

1.Finely chop celery, carrots, garlic, onion and water chestnuts in a food processor. Parts must be small and fairly uniform, but not liquid.

2.Mix ground pork and chopped vegetables in a large frying pan.

3.Cook over medium heat until the vegetables are soft and the pork is no longer pink.

4.Turn up the heat and let the moisture evaporate, then add the peanut sauce and cook for another 5 minutes before removing it from the heat.

5.While cooking the pork mixture, preheat the oven to 175 ° C (350 ° F).

6.Press a wonton wrap into each cup of a mini muffin pan, with flared edges on the sides.

7.Place a spoonful of the meat mixture in each cup.

8.Bake in the preheated oven for about 12 minutes or until the outer envelopes are crispy and golden brown.

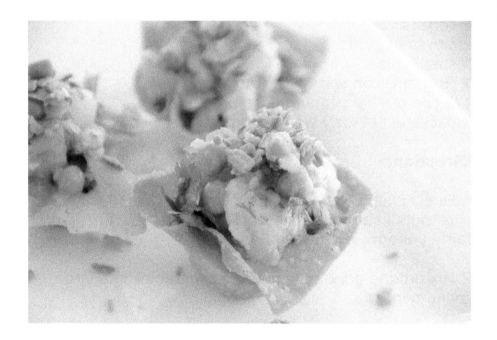

Sesame Stick Snacks

Preparation Time: 15 minutes
Cooking Time: 15 minutes
Servings: 10

Ingredients:

2 cups biscuit baking mix
2/3 cup heavy cream
1/4 cup butter, melted
1 1/2 tablespoons sesame seeds

Directions:

1.Preheat the oven to 220 ° C. Lightly grease 2 baking trays.

2.Mix the dough mixture and the cream; mix for 30 seconds.

3.Turn the dough on a lightly floured surface and knead 10 times. Roll the dough into a 5 x 10- inch rectangle.

4.Cut the dough into 1/2 inch wide strips.

5.Place the strips on prepared baking trays. Brush the strips with melted butter and sprinkle with sesame seeds.

6.Bake in the preheated oven for 15 minutes, until golden brown.

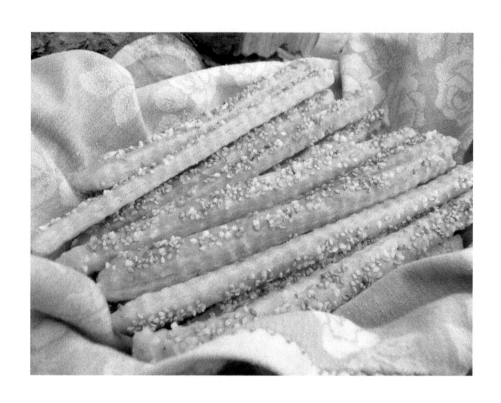

Shawn's Study Snacks
Preparation Time: 10 minutes
Cooking Time: 10 minutes
Servings: 60

Ingredients:

3 bananas, pureed
3/4 cup butter
1 egg
1 cup of white sugar
1/4 cup of packaged brown sugar
1 teaspoon baking powder
2 1/2 cups flour
1/4 teaspoon ground nutmeg
1/2 teaspoon ground cinnamon
1 1/2 cups oatmeal
3/4 cup chopped walnuts
1/2 cup raisins (optional)

Directions:

1.Preheat the oven to 175 ° C (350 ° F).
Mix in order, making sure the butter or margarine is well absorbed. More flour can be added if needed.

2.Spoon soup on a greased baking sheet. Bake for 10 minutes or until the edges are light brown.

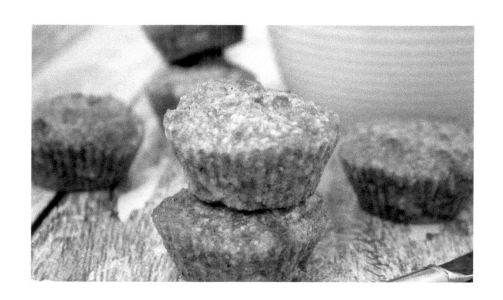

Pistachio Arugula Salad

Preparation Time: 20 minutes
Cooking Time: 0 minutes
Servings: 6

Ingredients:

¼ Cup Olive Oil
6 Cups Kale, Chopped Rough
2 Cups arugula
½ Teaspoon Smoked Paprika
2 Tablespoons Lemon Juice, Fresh
1/3 Cup Pistachios, Unsalted & Shelled
6 Tablespoons Parmesan, Grated

Directions:

1.Get out a large bowl and combine your oil, lemon juice, kale and smoked paprika.

2.Massage it into the leaves for about fifteen seconds. You then need to allow it to sit for ten minutes.

3.Mix everything together before serving with grated cheese on top.

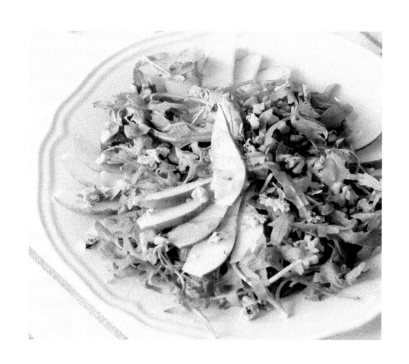

Potato Salad
Preparation Time: 10 minutes
Cooking Time: 15 minutes
Servings: 6

Ingredients:

2 lbs. Golden Potatoes, Cubed in 1 Inch Pieces
3 Tablespoons Olive Oil
3 tablespoons Lemon Juice, Fresh
1 Tablespoon Olive Brine
¼ Teaspoon Sea Salt, Fine
½ Cup Olives, Sliced
1 Cup Celery, Sliced
2 Tablespoons Oregano, Fresh
2 Tablespoons Mint Leaves, Fresh & Chopped

Directions:

1.Get out a medium saucepan and put your potatoes in cold water. The water should be earn inch above your potatoes.

2.Set it over high heat and bring it to a boil before turning the heat down. You want to turn it down to medium-low.

3.Allow it to cook for twelve to fifteen more minutes. The potatoes should be tender when you pierce them with a fork.

4.Get out a small bowl and whisk your oil, lemon juice, olive brine and salt together.

5.Drain your potatoes using a colander and transfer it to a serving bowl. Pour in three tablespoons of dressing over your potatoes, and mix well with oregano, and min along with the remaining dressing.

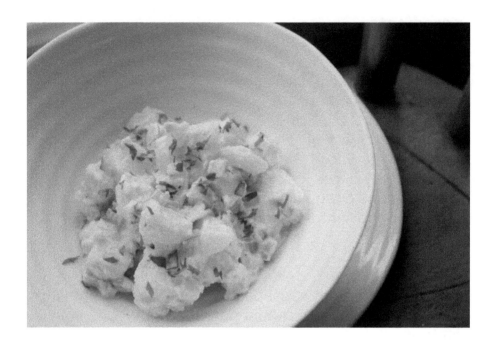

Raisin Rice Pilaf

Preparation Time: 7 minutes
Cooking Time: 8 minutes
Servings: 5

Ingredients:

1 Tablespoon Olive Oil
1 Teaspoon Cumin
1 Cup Onion, Chopped
½ Cup Carrot, Shredded
½ Teaspoon Cinnamon
2 Cups Instant Brown Rice
1 ¾ Cup Orange Juice
1 Cup Golden Raisins
¼ Cup Water
½ Cup Pistachios, Shelled
Fresh Chives, Chopped for Garnish

Directions:

1.Place a medium saucepan over medium-high heat before adding in your oil.

2.Add n your onion, and stir often so it doesn't burn.

3.Cook for about five minutes and then add in your cumin, cinnamon and carrot. Cook for about another minute.

4.Add in your orange juice, water and rice. Bring it all to a boil before covering your saucepan.

5.Turn the heat down to medium-low and then allow it to simmer for six to seven minutes. Your rice should be cooked all the way through, and all the liquid should be absorbed.

6.Stir in your pistachios, chives and raisins. Serve warm.

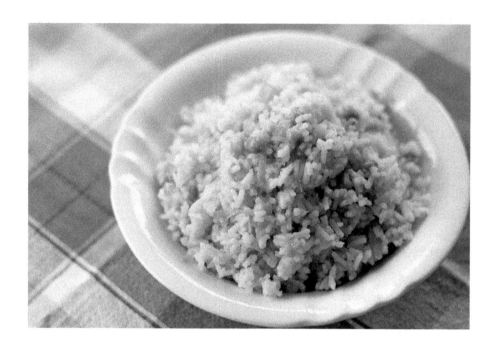

Lebanesen Delight

Preparation Time: 10 minutes
Cooking Time: 15 minutes
Servings: 5

Ingredients:

1 Tablespoon Olive Oil
1 Cup Vermicelli (Can be Substituted for Thin Spaghetti) Broken into 1 to 1
½ inch Pieces
3 Cups Cabbage, Shredded
3 Cups Vegetable Broth, Low Sodium
½ Cup Water
1 Cup Instant Brown Rice
¼ Teaspoon Sea Salt, Fine
2 Cloves Garlic
¼ Teaspoon Crushed Red Pepper
½ Cup Cilantro Fresh & Chopped Lemon Slices to Garnish

Directions:

1.Get out a saucepan and then place it over medium-high heat.

2.Add in your oil and once it's hot you will need to add in your pasta.

3.Cook for three minutes or until your pasta is toasted. You will have to stir often in order to keep it from burning.

4.Add in your cabbage, cooking for another four minutes. Continue to stir often.

5.Add in your water and rice. Season with salt, red pepper and garlic before bringing it all to a boil over high heat. Stir, and then cover.

6.Once it's covered turn the heat down to medium-low. Allow it all to simmer for ten minutes.

7.Remove the pan from the burner and then allow it to sit without lifting the lid for five minutes. Take the garlic cloves out and then mash them using a fork.

8.Place them back in, and stir them into the rice. Stir in your cilantro as well and serve warm. Garnish with lemon wedges if desired.

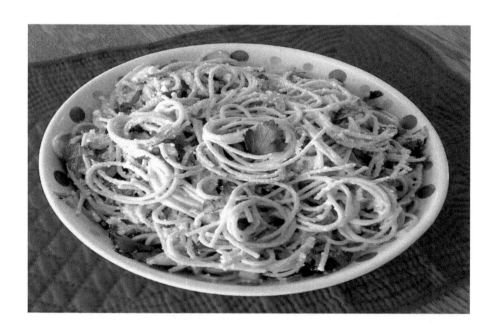

Mediterranean Sweet Potato

Preparation Time: 10 minutes
Cooking Time: 25 minutes
Servings: 4

Ingredients:

4 Sweet Potatoes
15 Ounce Can Chickpeas, Rinsed & Drained
½ Tablespoon Olive Oil
½ Teaspoon Cumin
½ Teaspoon Coriander
½ Teaspoon Cinnamon
1 Pinch Sea Salt, Fine
½ Teaspoon Paprika
¼ Cup Hummus
1 Tablespoon Lemon Juice, Fresh 2-3 Teaspoon Dill, Fresh
3 Cloves Garlic, Minced
Unsweetened Almond Milk as Needed

Directions:

1.Start by preheating your oven to 400, and then get out a baking sheet. Line it with foil.

2.Wash your sweet potatoes before halving them lengthwise.

3.Take your olive oil, cumin, chickpeas, coriander, sea salt and paprika on your baking sheet. Rub the sweet potatoes with olive oil, placing them face down over the mixture.

4.Roast for twenty to twenty-five minutes. They should become tender, and your chickpeas should turn a golden color.

5.Once it's in the oven, you can prepare your sauce. To do this mix your dill, lemon juice, hummus, garlic and a dash of almond milk. Mix well. Add more almond milk to thin as necessary. Adjust the seasoning if necessary.

6.Smash the insides of the sweet potato down, topping with chickpea mixture and sauce before serving.

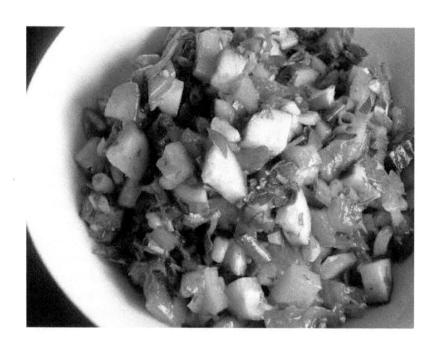

Flavorful Braised Kale

Preparation Time: 15 minutes
Cooking Time: 15 minutes
Servings: 6

Ingredients:

1 lb. Kale, Stems Removed & Chopped Roughly
1 Cup Cherry Tomatoes, Halved
2 Teaspoons Olive Oil
4 Cloves Garlic, Sliced Thin
½ Cup Vegetable Stock
¼ Teaspoon Sea Salt, Fine
1 Tablespoon Lemon Juice, Fresh
1/8 Teaspoon Black Pepper

Directions:

1.Start by heating your olive oil in a frying pan using medium heat, and add in your garlic. Sauté for a minute or two until lightly golden.

2.Mix your kale and vegetable stock with your garlic, adding it to your pan. Cover the pan and then turn the heat down to medium-low.

3.Allow it to cook until your kale wilts and part of your vegetable stock should be dissolved. It should take roughly five minutes.

4.Stir in your tomatoes and cook without a lid until your kale is tender, and then remove it from heat.

5.Mix in your salt, pepper and lemon juice before serving warm.

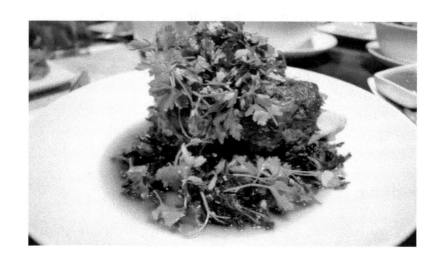

Bean Salad

Preparation Time: 15 minutes
Cooking Time: 5 minutes
Servings: 6

Ingredients:

1 Can Garbanzo Beans, Rinsed & Drained
2 Tablespoons Balsamic Vinegar
¼ Cup Olive Oil
4 Cloves Garlic, Chopped Fine
1/3 Cup Parsley, Fresh & Chopped
¼ Cup Olive Oil
1 Red Onion, Diced 6 Lettuce Leaves
½ Cup Celery, Chopped Fine/Black Pepper to Taste

Directions:

1.Make the vinaigrette dressing by whipping together your garlic, parsley, vinegar and pepper in a bowl.

2.Add the olive oil to this mixture and whisk before setting it aside.

3.Add in your onion and beans, and then pour your dressing on top. Toss until it's coated together and then cover it. Place it in the fridge until it's time to serve.

4.Place a lettuce leaf on the plate when serving and spoon the mixture in. garnish with celery.

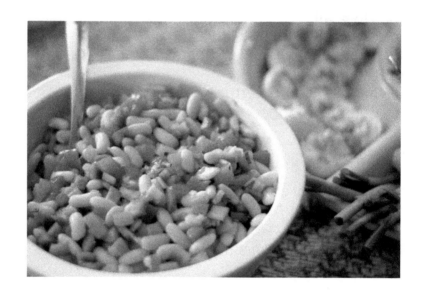

Basil Tomato Skewers

Preparation Time: 10 minutes
Cooking Time: 0 minutes
Servings: 2

Ingredients:

16 Mozzarella Balls, Fresh & Small
16 Basil Leaves, Fresh
16 Cherry Tomatoes Olive Oil to Drizzle
Sea Salt & Black Pepper to Taste

Directions:

1.Start by threading your basil, cheese and tomatoes together on small skewers.

2.Drizzle with oil before seasoning with salt and pepper.

3.Serve immediately.

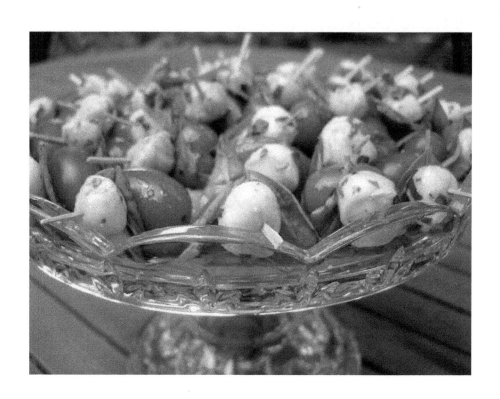

Olives with Feta

Preparation Time: 5 minutes
Cooking Time: 0 minutes
Servings: 4

Ingredients:

½ Cup Feta Cheese, Diced
1 Cup Kalamata Olives, Sliced & Pitted
2 Cloves Garlic, Sliced
2 Tablespoons Olive Oil
1 Lemon, Zested & Juiced
1 Teaspoon Rosemary, Fresh & Chopped Crushed Red
Pepper
Black Pepper to Taste

Directions:

1.Mix everything together and serve over crackers.

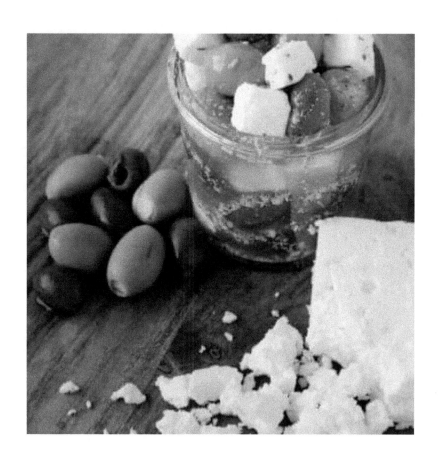

Black Bean Medley

Preparation Time: 5 minutes
Cooking Time: 0 minutes
Servings: 4

Ingredients:

4 Plum Tomatoes, Chopped
14.5 Ounces Black Beans, Canned & Drained
½ Red Onion, Sliced
¼ Cup Dill, Fresh & Chopped
1 Lemon, Juiced
2 Tablespoons Olive Oil
¼ Cup Feta Cheese, Crumbled
Sea Salt to Taste

Directions:

1.Mix everything in a bowl except for your feta and salt.
Top the beans with salt and feta.

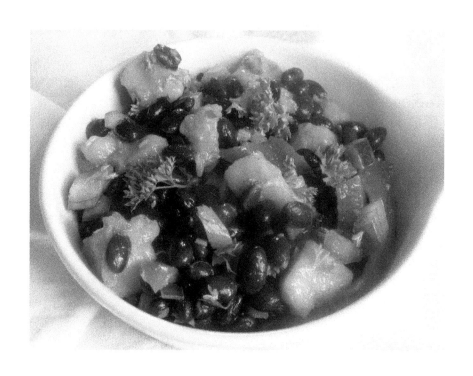

Spiced Popcorn

Preparation Time: 5 minutes
Cooking Time: 5 minutes
Servings: 4

Ingredients:

3 tablespoons olive oil
½ cup popcorn kernels Cooking spray
1 teaspoon garlic powder
1 teaspoon onion powder
½ teaspoon smoked paprika
½ teaspoon salt
⅛ Teaspoon cayenne pepper

Directions:

1.In a medium pot over medium-low heat, heat the olive oil.

2.Add 3 popcorn kernels, and when one of the kernels pops, add the rest.

3.Cover and shake the pot occasionally to prevent burning. Once fully popped, transfer the popcorn to a large bowl.

4.Spray the popcorn with cooking spray. Use clean hands to toss the popcorn, mixing it thoroughly.

5.In a small bowl, mix together the garlic powder, onion powder, paprika, salt, and cayenne.

6.Sprinkle the spice mix over the popcorn, and toss until the popcorn is thoroughly coated.

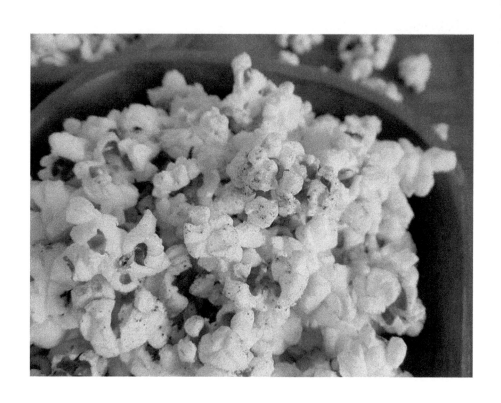

Baked Spinach Chips

Preparation Time: 5 minutes
Cooking Time: 15 minutes
Servings: 4

Ingredients:

Cooking spray
5 ounces baby spinach, washed and patted dry
2 tablespoons olive oil
1 teaspoon garlic powder
½ teaspoon salt
⅛ Teaspoon freshly ground black pepper

Directions:

1.Preheat the oven to 350°F. Coat two baking sheets with cooking spray.

2.Place the spinach in a large bowl. Add the olive oil, garlic powder, salt, and pepper, and toss until evenly coated.

3.Spread the spinach in a single layer on the baking sheets. Bake for 12 to 15 minutes, until the spinach leaves are crisp and slightly browned.

4.Store spinach chips in a resalable container at room temperature for up to 1 week.

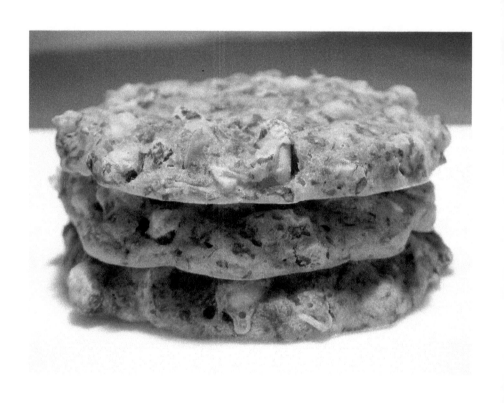

Peanut Butter Yogurt Dip with Fruit

Preparation Time: 10 minutes
Cooking Time: 0 minutes
Servings: 4

Ingredients:

1cup nonfat vanilla Greek yogurt
2tablespoons natural creamy peanut butter
2teaspoons honey
1pear, cored and sliced
1 apple, cored and sliced
1 banana, sliced

Directions:

1.In a medium bowl, whisk together the yogurt, peanut butter, and honey.

2.Serve the dip with the fruit on the side.

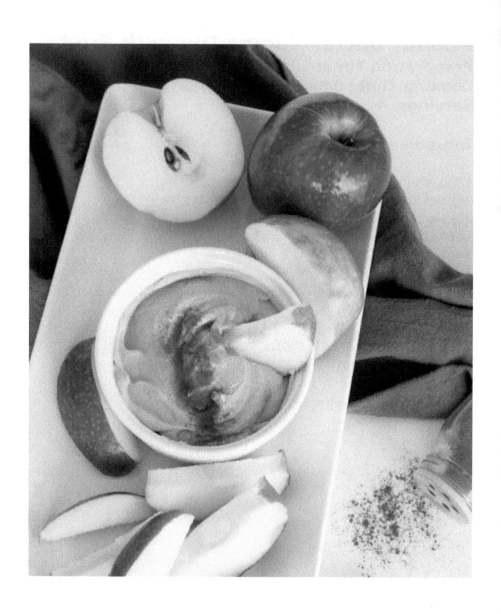

Snickerdoodle Pecans

Preparation Time: 10 minutes
Cooking Time: 15 minutes
Servings: 8

Ingredients:

Cooking spray
1½ cups raw pecans
2 tablespoons brown sugar
2 tablespoons 100% maple syrup
½ teaspoon ground cinnamon
½ teaspoon vanilla extract
⅛ Teaspoon salt

Directions:

1.Preheat the oven to 350°F. Line a baking sheet with parchment paper and coat with cooking spray.

2.In a medium bowl, place the pecans. Add the brown sugar, maple syrup, cinnamon, vanilla, and salt, tossing to evenly coat.

3.Spread the pecans in a single layer on the prepared baking sheet. Bake for about 12 minutes, until pecans are slightly browned and fragrant.

4.Remove and set aside to cool for 10 minutes.

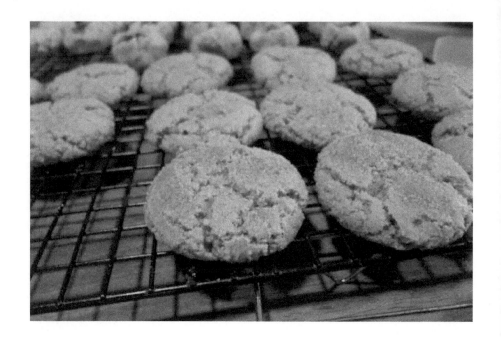

Almond-Stuffed Dates

Preparation Time: 5 minutes
Cooking Time: 0 minutes
Servings: 4

Ingredients:

20 raw almonds
20 pitted dates

Directions:

1.Place one almond into each of 20 dates.

2.Serve at room temperature.

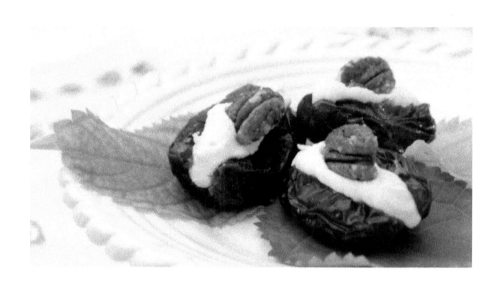

Peanut Butter Chocolate Chip Energy Bites

Preparation Time: 20 minutes
Cooking Time: 5 minutes
Servings: 12

Ingredients:

1 cup gluten-free old-fashioned oats
¾ cup natural creamy peanut butter
½ cup unsweetened coconut flakes
½ teaspoon vanilla extract
2 tablespoons honey
¼ cup dark chocolate chips

Directions:

1.Preheat the oven to 350°F. Line a baking sheet with parchment paper.

2.Spread the oats on the prepared baking sheet. Bake for 5 minutes, until the oats are browned. Remove from the oven, and set aside to cool for 5 minutes.

3.In a food processor or blender, add the oats, peanut butter, coconut, vanilla, and honey. Blend until smooth.

3.Transfer the batter into a medium bowl, and fold in the chocolate chips. Spoon out a tablespoon of batter.

4.Use clean hands to roll into a 2-inch ball, and place on the baking sheet. Repeat for the remaining batter, making a total of 12 balls.

5.Place the baking sheet in the refrigerator to allow the bites to set, at least 15 minutes.

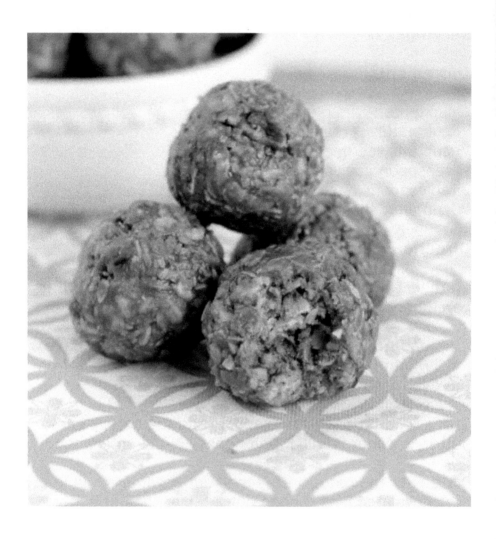

No-Cook Pistachio-Cranberry Quinoa Bites

Preparation Time: 15 minutes
Cooking Time: 0 minutes
Servings: 12

Ingredients:

½ cup quinoa
¾ cup natural almond butter
¾ cup gluten-free old-fashioned oats
2 tablespoons honey
⅛ Teaspoon salt
¼ cup unsalted shelled pistachios, roughly chopped
¼ cup dried cranberries

Directions:

1.In a blender, add the quinoa and blend until it turns into a flour consistency. Add the almond butter, oats, honey, and salt, and blend until smooth.

2.Transfer the mixture into a medium bowl, and gently fold in the pistachios and cranberries.

3.Spoon out a tablespoon of the batter. Use clean hands to roll into a 2-inch ball, and place into a container.
4.Repeat for the remaining batter, making a total of 12 balls.

5.Place the container in the refrigerator to allow the bites to set, at least 15 minutes.

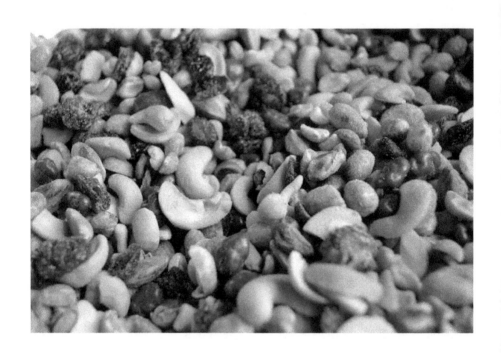

No-Bake Honey-Almond Granola Bars

Preparation Time: 15 minutes
Cooking Time: 0 minutes
Servings: 8

Ingredients:

Cooking spray
1 cup pitted dates
¼ cup honey
¾ cup natural creamy almond butter
¾ cup gluten-free rolled oats
2 tablespoons raw almonds, chopped
2 tablespoons pumpkin seeds

Directions:

1.Line an 8-by-8-inch baking dish with parchment paper, and coat the paper with cooking spray.

2.In a food processor or blender, add the dates and blend until they reach a pastelike consistency. Add the honey, almond butter, and oats, and blend until well combined. Transfer the mixture to a medium bowl.

3.Add the almonds and pumpkin seeds, and gently fold until well combined. Spoon the mixture into the prepared baking dish. Spread the mixture evenly, using clean fingers to push down the mixture so it is compact.

4.Cover with plastic wrap and refrigerate until the bars set, 1 to 2 hours. Remove from the refrigerator and cut into 8 bars.

5.Carefully remove each bar from the baking dish, and wrap individually in plastic wrap. Place bars in the refrigerator until ready to grab and go.

Cottage Cheese–Filled Avocado

Preparation Time: 5 minutes
Cooking Time: 0 minutes
Servings: 4

Ingredients:

½ cup low-fat cottage cheese
¼ cup cherry tomatoes, quartered
2 avocados, halved and pitted
4 teaspoons pumpkin seeds
¼ teaspoon salt
⅛ Teaspoon freshly ground black pepper

Directions:

1.In a small bowl, mix together the cottage cheese and tomatoes.

2.Spoon 2 tablespoons of the cheese-tomato mixture onto each of the avocado halves.

3.Top each with 1 teaspoon of pumpkin seeds, and sprinkle with the salt and pepper.

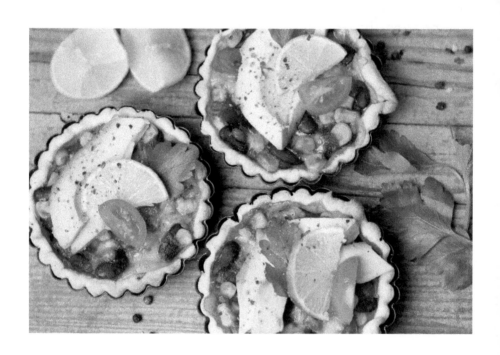

Avocado Toast with Balsamic Glaze

Preparation Time: 5 minutes
Cooking Time: 10 minutes
Servings: 2

Ingredients:

¼ cup balsamic vinegar
1 tablespoon brown sugar
1 ripe avocado, halved and pitted
2 slices 100% whole-wheat bread, toasted
5 cherry tomatoes, halved
⅛ Teaspoon salt
⅛ Teaspoon freshly ground black pepper

Directions:

1.In a small saucepan over medium heat, heat the vinegar and brown sugar, stirring constantly, until the sugar dissolves.

2.Bring the mixture to a boil, lower heat, and simmer for about 10 minutes, until the vinegar is reduced by half and thickens.

3.Set aside to cool for 10 minutes.
Scoop out the flesh from each avocado half onto a slice of toasted bread.

4.Mash the avocado with a fork until it is flattened.

5.Top each slice of bread with 5 tomato halves, and sprinkle with the salt and pepper.

6.Drizzle about ½ tablespoon of the balsamic glaze on each avocado toast.

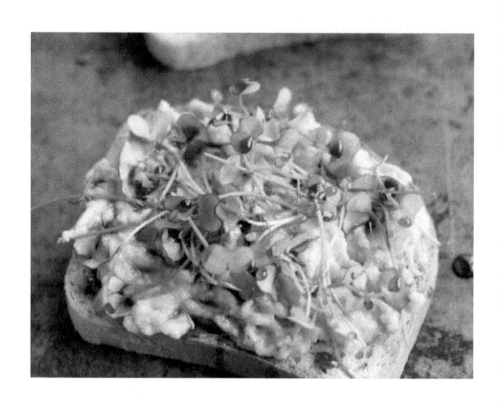

Lightning Source UK Ltd.
Milton Keynes UK
UKHW020639230421
382498UK00009B/481